American Red Cross

OXYGEN ADMINISTRATION

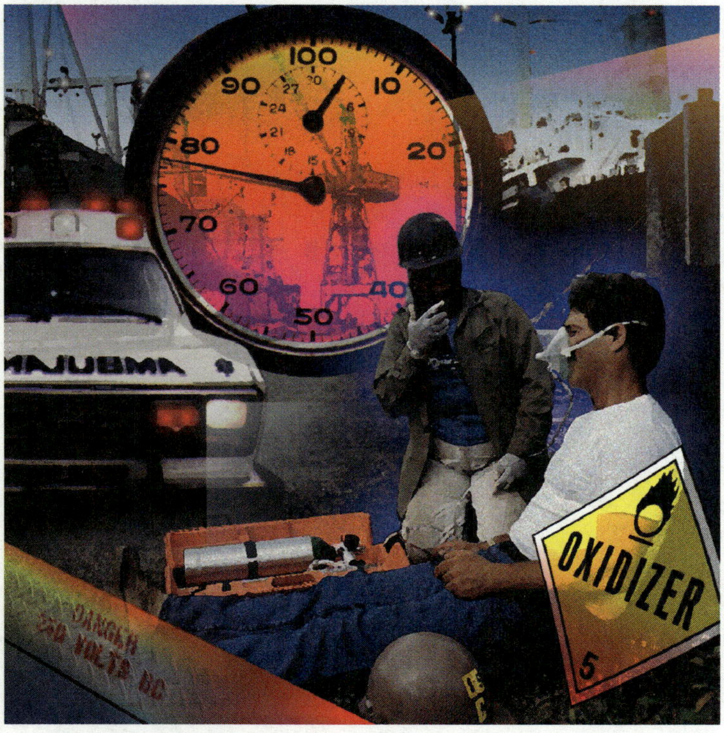

Mosby Lifeline
St. Louis Baltimore Boston Chicago London Philadelphia Sydney Toronto

Mosby Lifeline
Dedicated to Publishing Excellence

A Mosby Lifeline imprint of Mosby–Year Book, Inc.

Printed in the United States of America

Mosby Lifeline
Mosby–Year Book, Inc.
11830 Westline Industrial Drive
St. Louis, Missouri 63146

ISBN 0-8016-7276-7

93 94 95 96 97 CL/CD/CA 9 8 7 6 5 4 3 2 1

Dedicated to the thousands
of first responders who give unselfishly of
themselves to save lives.

Oxygen Administration

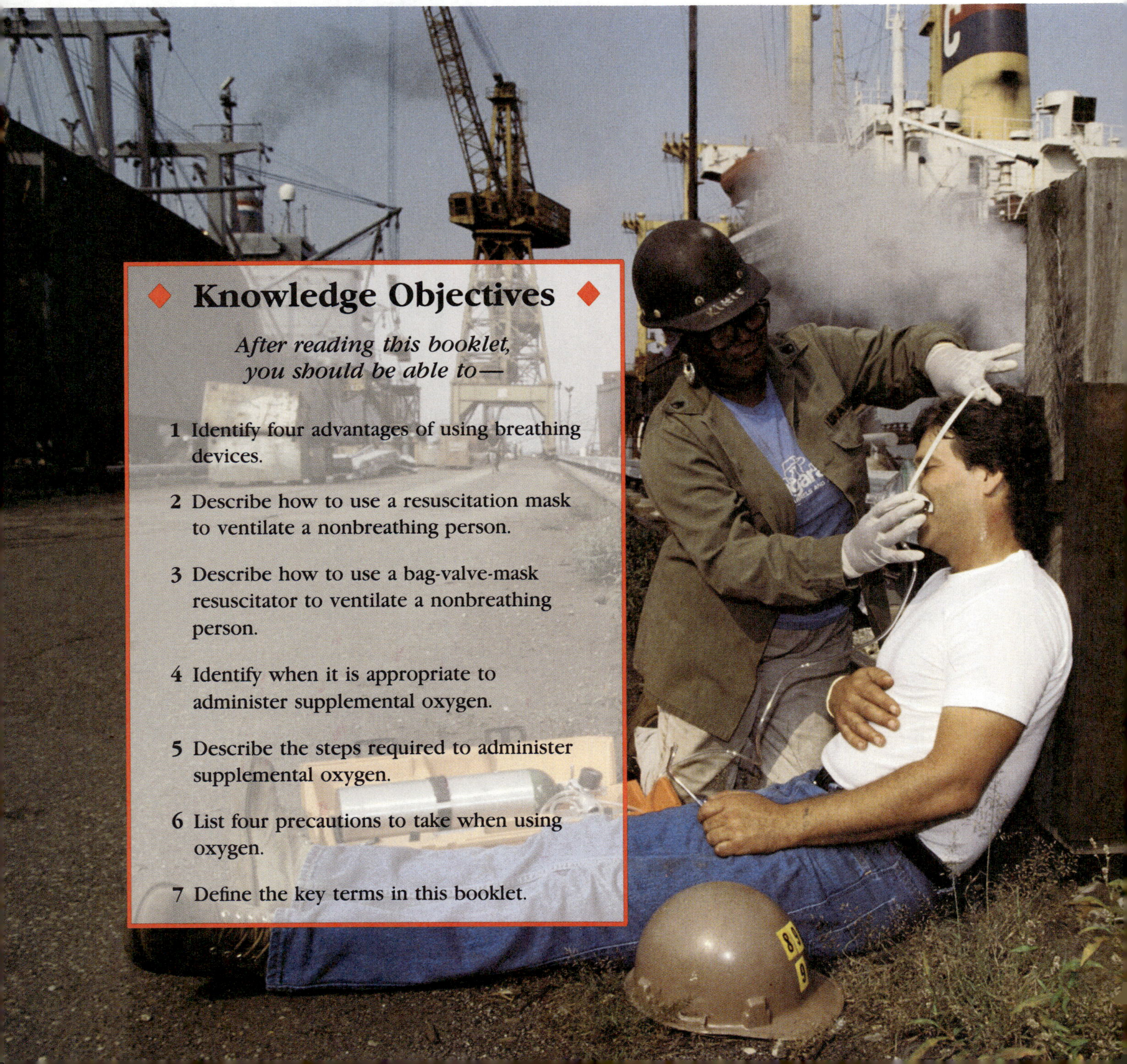

Knowledge Objectives

After reading this booklet, you should be able to—

1. Identify four advantages of using breathing devices.
2. Describe how to use a resuscitation mask to ventilate a nonbreathing person.
3. Describe how to use a bag-valve-mask resuscitator to ventilate a nonbreathing person.
4. Identify when it is appropriate to administer supplemental oxygen.
5. Describe the steps required to administer supplemental oxygen.
6. List four precautions to take when using oxygen.
7. Define the key terms in this booklet.

◆ Skill Objectives ◆

After reading this booklet and completing the activities, you should be able to—

1 Demonstrate on a manikin how to use a resuscitation mask to ventilate a nonbreathing person.

2 Demonstrate how to prepare the equipment to administer oxygen to a breathing or a nonbreathing person.

3 Make appropriate decisions about care when given an example of an emergency in which a person is having difficulty breathing.

◆ Key Terms ◆

Bag-valve-mask (BVM) resuscitator: A handheld ventilation device, consisting of a self-inflating bag, a one-way valve, and a face mask; can be used with or without supplemental oxygen.

Breathing devices: Devices used to help with ventilation.

Flowmeter: A device used to regulate in liters per minute (lpm) the amount of oxygen administered to a person.

Nasal cannula: A device used to administer oxygen through the nostrils to a breathing person.

Oxygen cylinder: A steel or alloy cylinder that contains 100 percent oxygen under high pressure.

Oxygen delivery device: A device used to administer oxygen from an oxygen cylinder to a person.

Pressure regulator: A device attached to an oxygen cylinder that reduces the delivery pressure of oxygen to a safe level.

Resuscitation mask: A pliable, dome-shaped device that fits over the nose and mouth, used to administer oxygen and assist with rescue breathing.

Supplemental oxygen: Additional oxygen provided to help resuscitate a person.

Ventilation: The process of providing oxygen to the lungs through rescue breathing or by other means.

INTRODUCTION

A 45-year-old man is experiencing chest pain. He states that it started about 30 minutes ago as a mild, squeezing sensation. Now the pain is severe and he is gasping for breath. You recognize that these signs and symptoms suggest a serious condition. While waiting for an ambulance to arrive, you do what you can for the person. You help him get into the most comfortable position and ask him to remain still. You open a nearby window to circulate fresh air into the stuffy room.

▼ ▼ ▼

You are called to assist a co-worker with an unknown medical emergency. You find a 60-year-old unconscious woman who is not breathing. You know what must be done and begin rescue breathing.

What do both of these situations have in common? Both are examples of situations in which **breathing devices** such as a resuscitation mask and supplemental oxygen would have been desirable and could have enhanced the care you were providing. Such devices can contribute significantly to the survival and recovery of a seriously ill or injured person.

Airway management is critical in life-threatening situations. In this booklet, you learn when and how to use various breathing devices to increase the effectiveness of the airway management you give a person who is injured or has suddenly become ill.

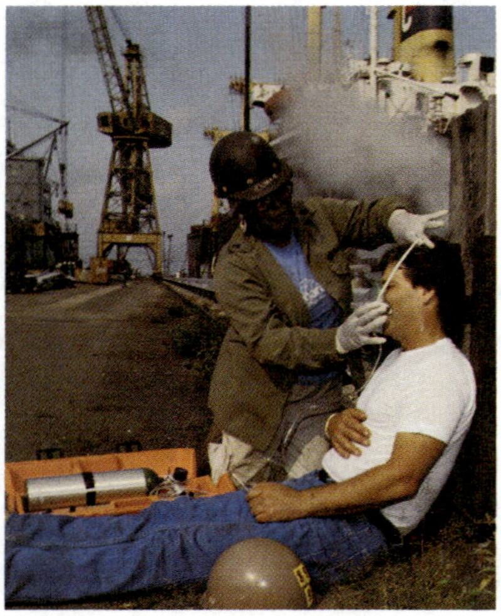

BREATHING DEVICES

Many different breathing devices are commonly used in the prehospital setting. Which breathing devices are routinely available to you will depend on your local standards and protocols. This booklet focuses on those breathing devices that you are likely to have immediately available or be asked to assist with in providing care. It is important to remember that *you should not delay care because a specific breathing device is not available.* Instead, you should start basic care, adding any breathing devices when they become available.

Breathing devices include resuscitation masks, bag-valve-mask resuscitators, and oxygen. In general, they provide several advantages. They can help you—

- Maintain an open airway.
- Perform rescue breathing.
- Limit the potential for disease transmission.
- Increase the oxygen concentration in a person's bloodstream.

◆ Resuscitation Masks

One of the most readily available, simple breathing devices is the **resuscitation mask.** Resuscitation masks are pliable, dome-shaped devices that fit over a person's mouth and nose, aiding **ventilation** (providing oxygen to the lungs). Several types of resuscitation masks are available, varying in size, shape, and features (Fig. 1).

Resuscitation masks offer you several advantages. These include—

- Increasing the flow of air to the lungs by permitting air to travel through a person's mouth and nose at the same time.
- Providing an adequate seal for ventilation, even when a person has facial injuries.
- Providing an effective and easily accessible alternative to other methods of ventilation, such as mouth-to-mouth or mouth-to-nose breathing or bag-valve-mask resuscitation.
- Permitting easy delivery of supplemental oxygen to either a breathing or a nonbreathing person.
- Reducing the possibility of disease transmission by providing a barrier between the rescuer and the victim.

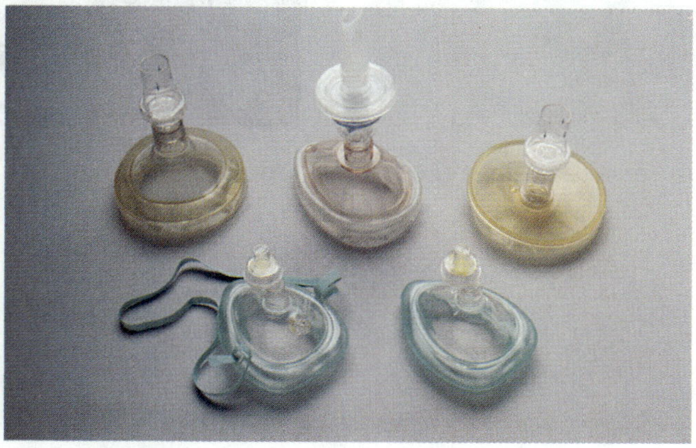

Figure 1
Resuscitation masks vary in size, shape, and features.

Selecting a resuscitation mask

For a resuscitation mask to be most effective, it should meet the following criteria:

- Be made of a transparent, pliable material that allows you to make a tight seal on the person's face when you perform rescue breathing or supply supplemental oxygen
- Have a one-way valve for releasing a person's exhaled air
- Have a standard 15-mm or 22-mm coupling assembly (the diameter of the opening that receives the one-way valve)
- Have an inlet for the delivery of supplemental oxygen
- Work well under a variety of environmental conditions such as extreme heat or cold
- Be easy to assemble and use

Figure 2 shows the features of an effective resuscitation mask.

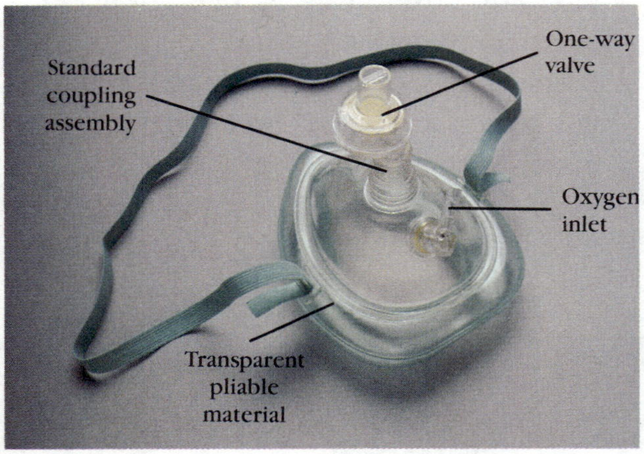

Figure 2 A resuscitation mask should meet specific criteria.

Using a resuscitation mask

When using a resuscitation mask during rescue breathing, begin by attaching the one-way valve to the mask. Next, place the mask so that it covers the person's mouth and nose. Position one rim of the mask between the lower lip and chin. The opposite end of the mask should cover the nose. Figure 3 shows how to assemble and position the resuscitation mask.

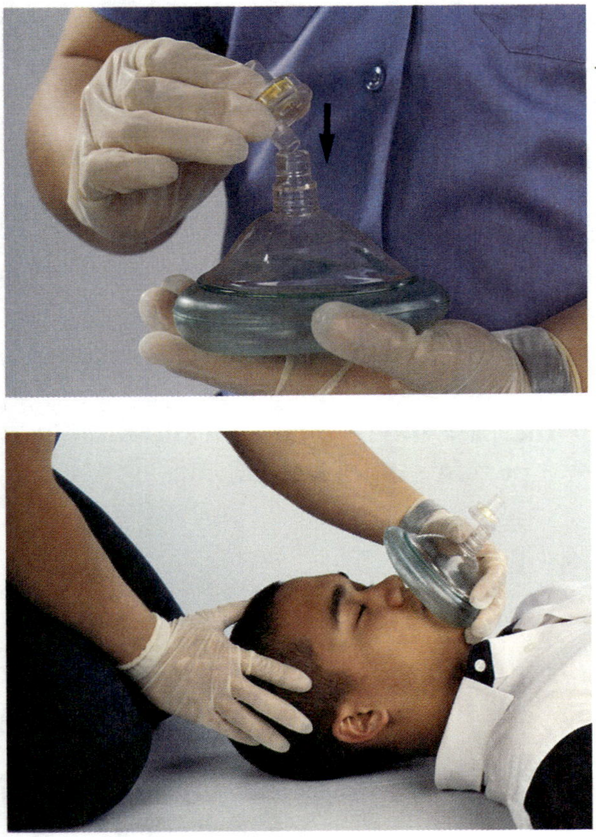

A

B

Figure 3 To use a resuscitation mask, **A,** begin by attaching the one-way valve to the mask. **B,** Position the mask to cover the mouth and nose.

When you use a resuscitation mask to give rescue breathing, you must maintain a good seal to prevent air from leaking at the edges of the mask. Use both hands to hold the mask in place and to maintain an open airway. You do this by following three steps. They involve—

- Tilting the person's head back.
- Lifting the jaw upward.
- Keeping the person's mouth open.

Figure 4 shows two methods for using a resuscitation mask.

If you suspect the victim has a head or spine injury, use the two-handed jaw thrust technique without tilting the head back. This technique can also be used with a resuscitation mask (Fig. 5). However, because the success of this technique depends on one's hand size and strength, some people will find it difficult to perform a two-handed jaw thrust using a resuscitation mask.

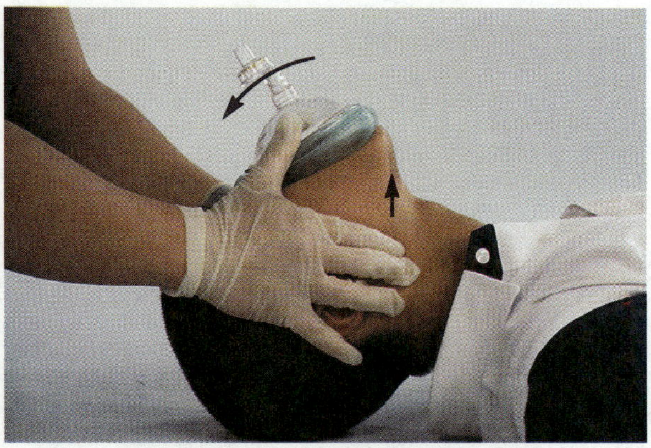

A

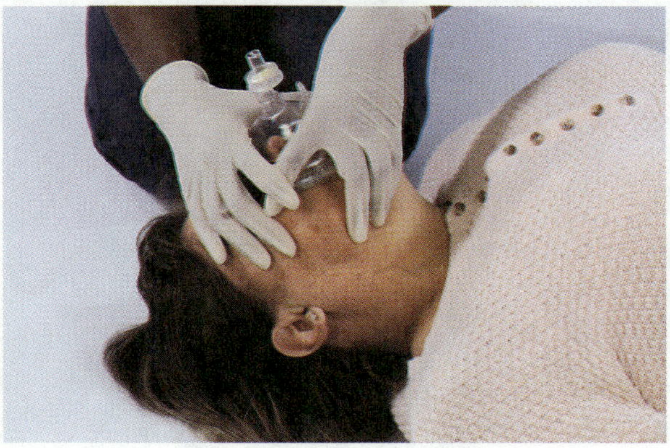

B

Figure 4 **A**, Tilt the head back, and lift the jaw to open the airway. **B**, Holding the mask from the side is an alternative method for using a resuscitation mask, for example, during one-rescuer CPR.

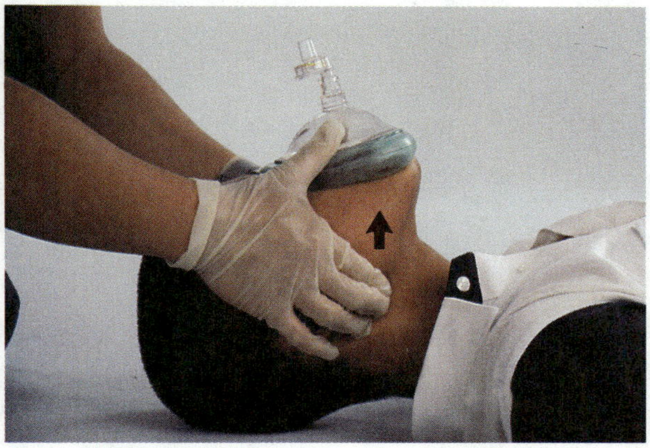

Figure 5 If you suspect a head or spine injury, lift the jaw, but do not tilt the head back.

◆ Bag-Valve-Mask Resuscitators

There may be times when you will have a bag-valve-mask resuscitator available or be asked to assist with one. A **bag-valve-mask (BVM) resuscitator** is a hand-held device, like the resuscitation mask, primarily used to ventilate a nonbreathing person. It is also used to assist ventilation of a person who is in respiratory distress.

The device has three main components: a bag, valve, and mask. The bag is self-inflating. Once compressed, it reinflates automatically. The one-way valve allows air to move from the bag to the victim but prevents the victim's exhaled air from entering the bag. The mask is similar to the resuscitation masks described earlier in this chapter. An oxygen reservoir bag should be attached to the BVM when supplemental oxygen is administered (Fig. 6).

The principle of the BVM is simple. By placing the mask on the victim's face and squeezing the bag, you open the one-way valve, forcing air into the victim's lungs. When you release the bag, the valve closes and air from the atmosphere refills the bag. At approximately the same time, the victim exhales. This exhaled air is diverted into the atmosphere through the closed one-way valve.

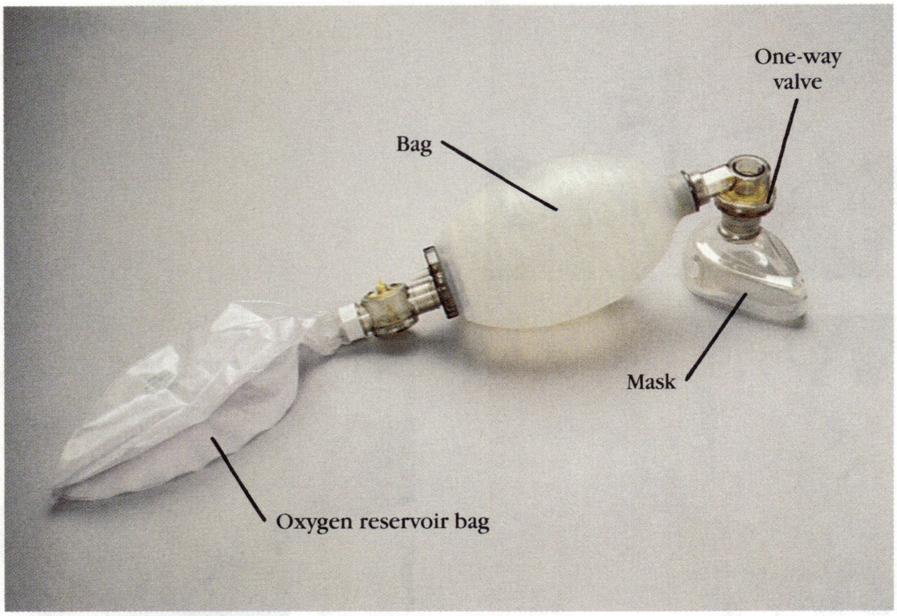

Figure 6 A bag-valve-mask (BVM) resuscitator consists of a bag, valve, and mask. An oxygen reservoir bag should be attached at the end of the bag when delivering supplemental oxygen.

Using a bag-valve-mask resuscitator

In the hands of a well-practiced rescuer, the bag-valve-mask (BVM) resuscitator is effective. But studies have shown that without consistent practice, single rescuers have a difficult time maintaining a tight enough seal and also maintaining an open airway for effective ventilation. For this reason, it is best if a BVM is used by two rescuers when possible.

When two rescuers are using a BVM, one rescuer positions the mask and opens the victim's airway. This is done in the same way as previously described for resuscitation masks. While the first rescuer maintains a tight seal with the mask on the victim's face (Fig. 7, *A*), the second rescuer provides ventilations by squeezing the bag until the victim's chest rises (Fig. 7, *B*). The bag should always be squeezed smoothly, not forcefully. This two-person technique is preferred because one rescuer can maintain an open airway and a tight mask seal, while a second rescuer can provide ventilations.

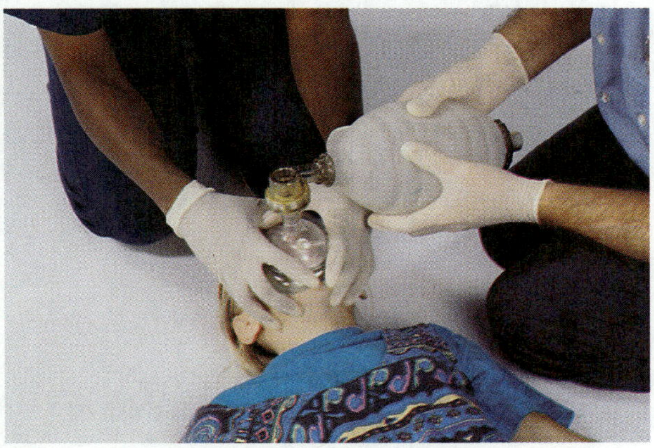

A

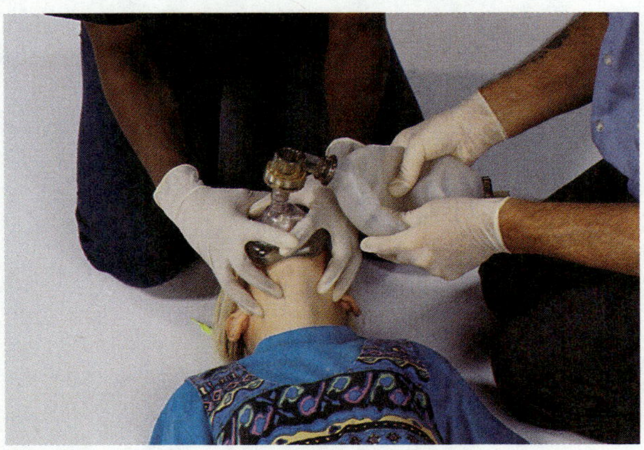

B

Figure 7 **A,** Position the mask over the victim's mouth and nose. Hold it in place as you would a resuscitation mask. **B,** Second rescuer squeezes the bag slowly until the chest rises.

If you must use a bag-valve-mask resuscitator alone, begin by assembling the bag, valve, and mask. Next, position the mask so that it covers the victim's mouth and nose in the same way previously described for resuscitation masks. Open the airway. With one hand, hold the mask in place by making a "C-clamp" with your index finger and thumb around the mask. Maintain an open airway using your other fingers to lift the jaw. You can use your knees to help hold the victim's head in this tilted position.

With one hand, press down on the mask to maintain a tight seal and help open the victim's mouth. With your other hand, squeeze the bag slowly until the victim's chest rises (Fig. 8). People with small hands or poor grip strength may find it necessary to compress the bag against their thigh to adequately ventilate the victim.

Advantages and disadvantages

Using the bag-valve-mask resuscitator has distinct advantages and disadvantages.

Advantages:

- It delivers a higher concentration of oxygen than that delivered during mouth-to-mouth or mouth-to-mask rescue breathing.
- It limits the potential for disease transmission.
- It is very effective when used by two rescuers.

Disadvantages:

- It is not an easy one-person skill to master.
- Without regular practice, you cannot stay proficient.
- It may take longer to assemble than other breathing devices.
- It is not a device readily available to you.

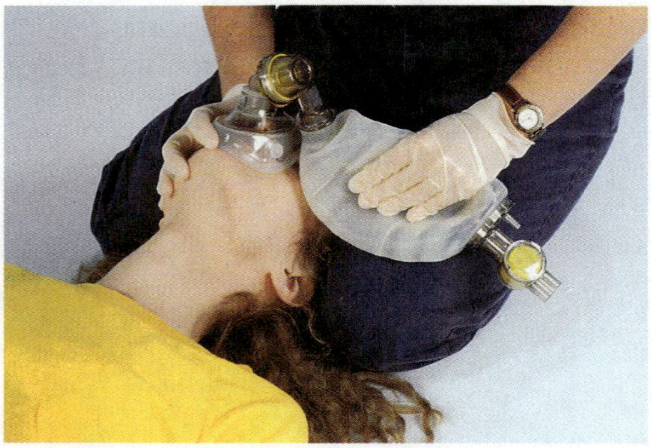

Figure 8 Compressing the bag against the thigh is a one-rescuer technique.

◆ Supplemental Oxygen

The normal concentration of oxygen in the air is approximately 21 percent. Under normal conditions, this is more than enough oxygen to sustain life. However, when serious injury or sudden illness occurs, the body does not function properly and can benefit from supplemental, or additional, oxygen. Without adequate oxygen, hypoxia will result. Hypoxia is a condition in which insufficient oxygen reaches the cells. When hypoxia occurs, it causes signs and symptoms that include increased breathing and heart rates, cyanosis (skin has a bluish color), changes in consciousness, restlessness, and chest pain.

For example, a person experiencing difficulty breathing and chest pain because of a heart attack or angina can have this pain and breathing discomfort reduced by the delivery of a higher concentration of oxygen. **Supplemental oxygen** delivered to the victim's lungs can help meet the increased demand for oxygen for all body tissues (Fig. 9).

If a heart attack victim suddenly suffers cardiac arrest, then you must use rescue breathing to force air into the victim's lungs. Whether you perform rescue breathing using the mouth-to-mouth or mouth-to-mask method, the oxygen concentration you deliver to the victim is only 16 percent. This is adequate to sus-

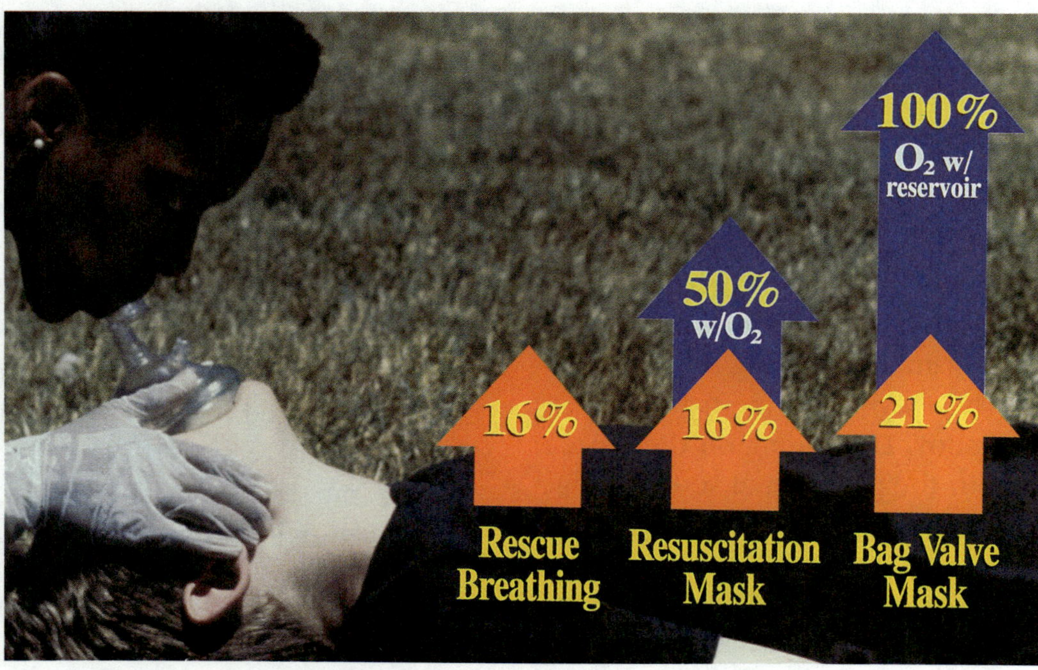

Figure 9 Breathing devices and supplemental oxygen can greatly increase the concentration of oxygen that a victim receives.

tain life in a healthy person. But, since chest compressions only circulate one-third normal blood flow under the best of conditions, body tissues are receiving only the bare minimum of oxygen required for short-term survival.

Using a bag-valve-mask resuscitator alone improves this situation only slightly, since it delivers atmospheric air (21 percent oxygen). A higher oxygen concentration helps to counter the effects of severe illness or injury to the body. Administering supplemental oxygen allows a substantially higher oxygen concentration, in some cases nearly 100 percent, to be delivered to the person.

To deliver supplemental oxygen, you must have—

- An oxygen cylinder.
- A pressure regulator with flowmeter.
- A delivery device.

Figure 10 shows an oxygen delivery system.

Oxygen cylinder

It is easy to recognize an **oxygen cylinder** because of its distinctive green color and yellow diamond marking that says *oxidizer.* These cylinders are made of steel or an alloy. Depending on their size, those used in the prehospital setting can hold between 350 and 625 liters of oxygen. These cylinders have internal pressures of approximately 2,000 pounds per square inch (psi).

Pressure regulator

The pressure inside the oxygen cylinder is far too great for a person to simply open the cylinder and administer the oxygen. Instead, a device must be attached to the cylinder to reduce the delivery pressure of the oxygen to a safe level. This regulating device is called a **pressure regulator.** The pressure regulator reduces the pressure from approximately 2,000 psi inside the cylinder to less than 70 psi.

A pressure regulator has a gauge that indicates how much pressure is in the cylinder. By checking the gauge, you can determine if a cylinder is full (2,000 psi), nearly empty (200 psi), or somewhere in between.

A pressure regulator has three metal prongs that fit into the valve at the top of the oxygen cylinder. The largest of these prongs must have a doughnut-shaped gasket, commonly called an "O-ring," attached. This gasket provides a tight seal between the oxygen cylinder and the pressure regulator.

Flowmeter

A **flowmeter** controls the amount of oxygen administered in liters per minute (lpm). Flowmeters normally deliver from 1 to 15 lpm, but some of the newer flowmeters can deliver as much as 25 lpm.

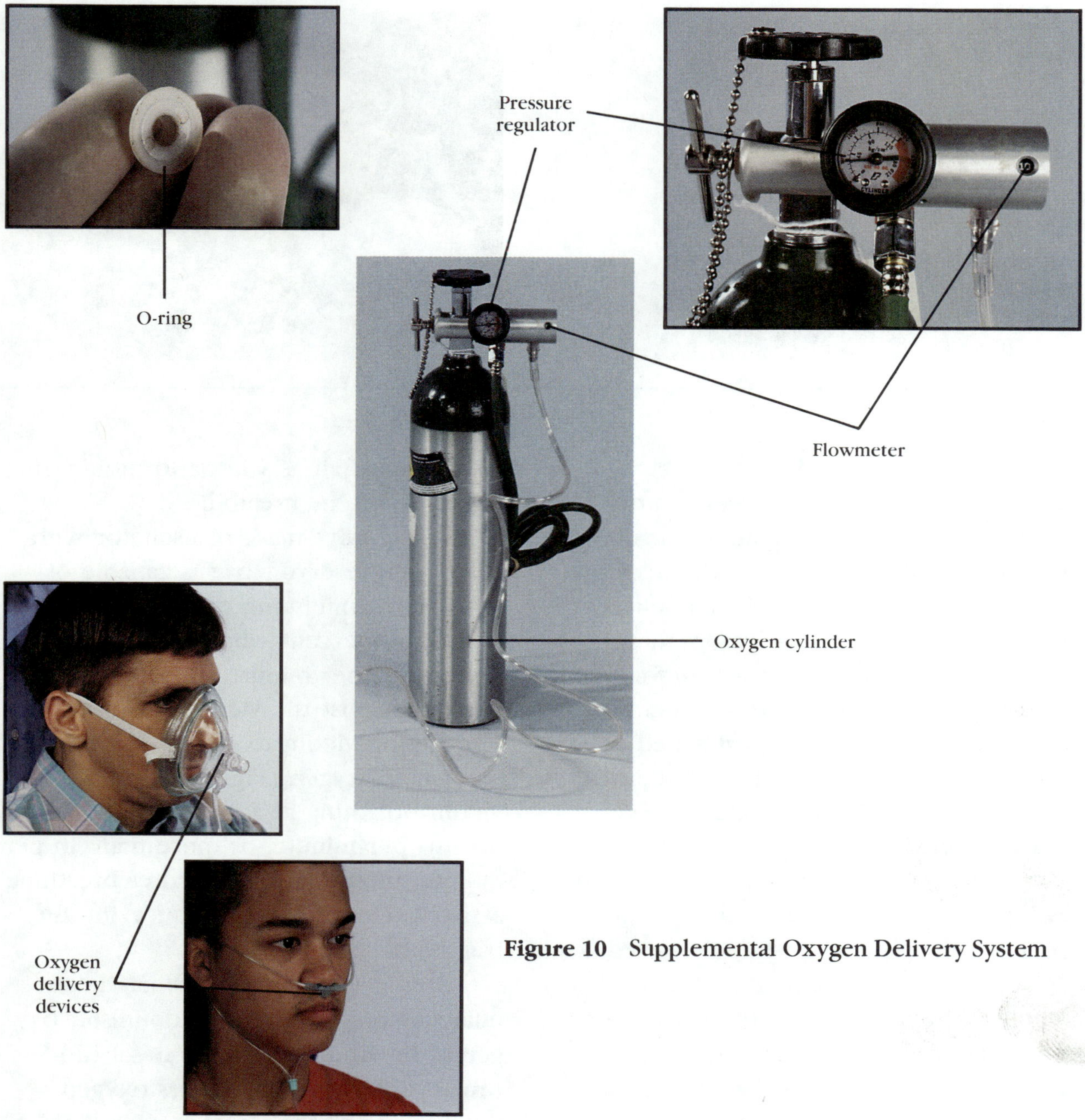

Figure 10 Supplemental Oxygen Delivery System

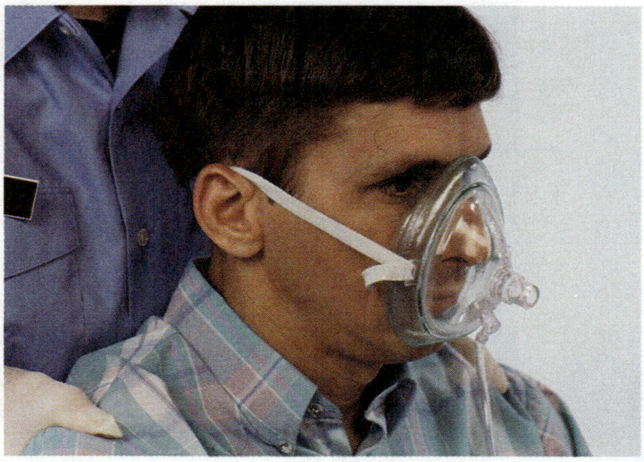

A

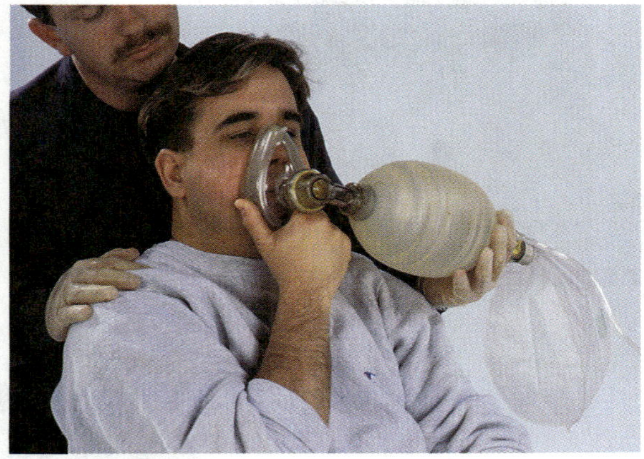

B

Oxygen delivery devices

Some **oxygen delivery devices** can deliver oxygen to either breathing or nonbreathing victims. Two devices, the resuscitation mask and the BVM, can deliver oxygen to both. For this reason, these devices are the most appropriate for you to use. Regardless of the device being used, a section of tubing is attached to the device at one end and to the flowmeter at the other end to create an oxygen-enriched environment for the victim.

A resuscitation mask is capable of delivering approximately 50 percent oxygen to a breathing person, when delivered at 6 or more liters per minute. This is substantially higher than the normal 21 percent that the victim is getting from the atmosphere. Some resuscitation masks have elastic straps attached to the mask. The elastic strap can be placed over the victim's head and tightened to help keep the mask securely in place (Fig. 11, *A*). If the mask does not have a strap, either you or the victim can hold it in place. When a resuscitation mask is used on a nonbreathing victim, it will deliver an oxygen concentration of approximately 35 percent. The oxygen concentration is reduced because oxygen mixes with your own exhaled air as you perform mouth-to-mouth rescue breathing.

The bag-valve-mask resuscitator with an oxygen reservoir bag is capable of supplying a minimum oxygen concentration of 90 percent when used at 10 or more liters per minute. The BVM can be held against the victim's face allowing a breathing victim to inhale the supplemental oxygen (Fig. 11, *B*). A victim breathing at a rate of less than 10 breaths per minute, or more than 30 per minute, should have his or her breathing assisted. This is done by squeezing the bag as the victim breathes.

Some devices, such as the nasal cannula, can only be used to administer oxygen to breathing victims. A **nasal cannula** is a device that delivers oxygen through the victim's nostrils (Fig. 11, *C*). It is a plastic tube with two small prongs that are inserted into the nose. The use of a nasal cannula is limited, since it is normally used at a flow rate of 1 to 4 lpm. Under these conditions, it delivers only a peak oxygen concentration of approximately 36 percent. Flow rates above 4 lpm are not commonly used because of the tendency to quickly dry out mucous membranes. This can cause nosebleeds and headaches.

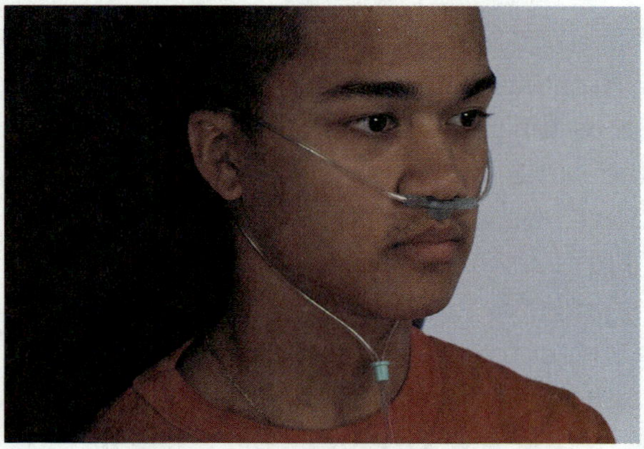

C

Figure 11 Common oxygen delivery devices include **A,** a resuscitation mask; **B,** a BVM; and **C,** a nasal cannula.

Because of its limitations, the nasal cannula is commonly used for people having only minor breathing difficulty. This device is not appropriate for victims experiencing serious respiratory distress, since they are generally breathing through their mouths and need a device that can supply a greater concentration of oxygen. In addition, the nasal cannula can be ineffective if the victim has a nasal airway obstruction, nasal injury, or bad cold causing blocked sinus passages. It should, however, be used if the victim cannot tolerate a mask over his or her face.

It is sometimes difficult to remember how many liters of oxygen to deliver. To eliminate confusion over how many liters of oxygen to deliver per minute, remember this general rule: *one to four and six or more.* For a nasal cannula, administering 1 to 4 lpm is appropriate. When using a mask that covers the victim's face, you can safely administer 6 or more liters per minute. Table 1 provides an overview of each of the delivery devices presented.

Table 1 Oxygen Delivery Devices

Device	Common flow rate	Oxygen concentration	Function
Nasal cannula	1-4 lpm	24-36 percent	Breathing victims only
Resuscitation mask	6+ lpm	35-55 percent	Breathing and nonbreathing victims
Bag-valve-mask resuscitator	10+ lpm	90+ percent	Breathing and nonbreathing victims

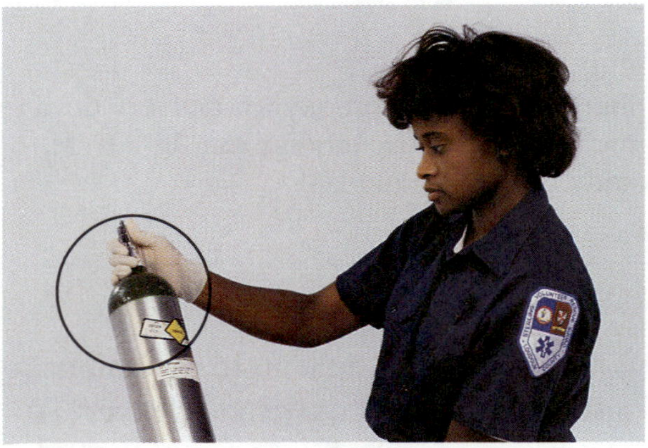

A

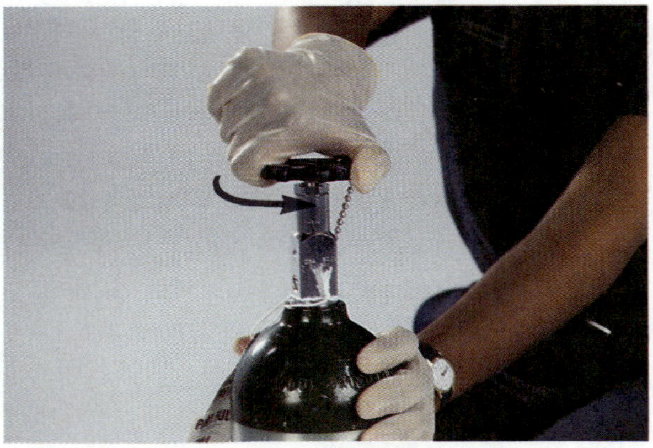

B

Figure 12 **A,** An oxygen cylinder is usually green, with a yellow diamond indicating oxygen. **B,** When preparing oxygen equipment, clear the cylinder valve by turning it counterclockwise.

Administering oxygen

Whether you are administering oxygen to a breathing or a nonbreathing person, the steps for preparing the equipment remain the same. Begin by examining the cylinder to be certain that it is labeled *oxygen* (Fig. 12, *A*). Next, check to see that the cylinder is full. Full cylinders come with a protective covering holding the plastic gasket (O-ring) in place. Remove this covering and save the gasket. Open the cylinder for 1 second (Fig. 12, *B*). This will remove any dirt or debris from the cylinder valve. Insert the gasket into the large opening of the cylinder (Fig. 13, *A*).

Next, examine the pressure regulator. Check to see that it is labeled *oxygen* pressure regulator (Fig. 13, *B*). Attach the pressure regulator to the cylinder, seating the three prongs inside the cylinder (Fig. 13, *C*). Hand tighten the screw until the regulator is snug (Fig. 13, *D*). Open the cylinder one full turn.

Check the pressure gauge to determine how much pressure is in the cylinder. A full cylinder should have approximately 2,000 psi. Attach the chosen delivery device to the oxygen port near the flowmeter. Some devices, such as the resuscitation mask and the BVM, require that you attach a section of the tubing between the flowmeter and the device. Other devices, such as the nasal cannula, have this section of tubing already attached.

Turn on the flowmeter to the desired flow rate (Fig. 14). Listen and feel to make sure that oxygen is flowing into your delivery device. Finally, place the delivery device on the victim.

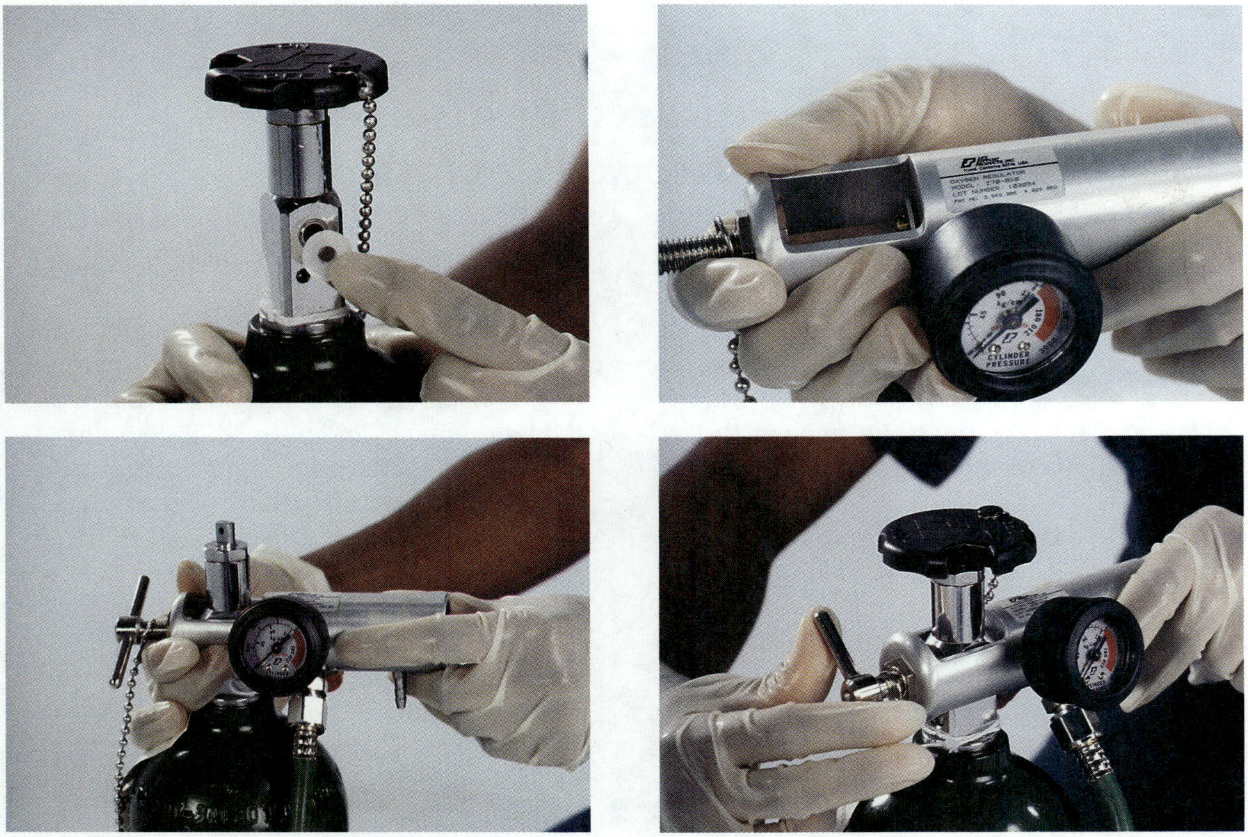

A B C D

Figure 13 To attach the pressure regulator to the oxygen cylinder, **A**, insert the gasket into the opening of the cylinder. **B,** Check to see that the pressure regulator is for use with oxygen. **C,** Seat the three prongs of the regulator inside the cylinder. **D,** Hand tighten the screw until the regulator is snug.

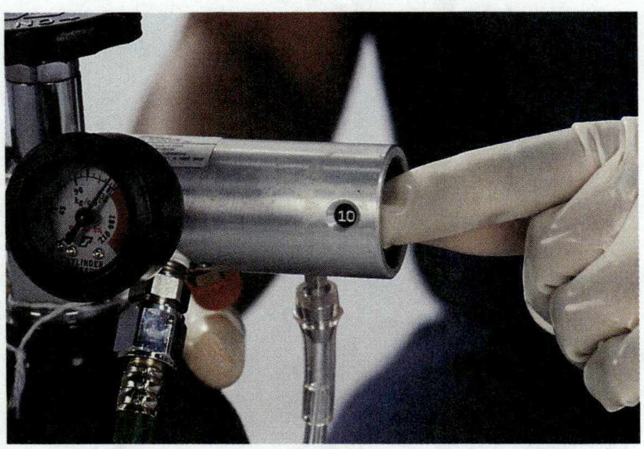

Figure 14 Turn the flowmeter clockwise to the desired flow rate.

Oxygen-Powered Resuscitators

The Controversy Continues

Oxygen-powered resuscitators, commonly called demand valves, have been the subject of controversy for several years. The points of controversy are whether these devices are as easy to use and whether they are as safe as other oxygen delivery devices. As the name *demand valve* implies, the victim can get oxygen on demand automatically.

A demand valve works in much the same way as a bag-valve-mask (BVM) resuscitator. However, instead of using a self-inflating bag as the ventilation source, it uses pressurized oxygen. The demand valve consists of a mask, a one-way valve, and an oxygen source. The mask is basically the same as that of the BVM unit. The one-way valve is designed to open and allow oxygen to flow to the breathing victim upon inhalation. The rescuer must depress a button to force oxygen into the lungs of a nonbreathing person. The use of the demand valve to ventilate a nonbreathing person is commonly called positive pressure resuscitation.

There are both advantages and disadvantages to using a demand valve. Advantages include delivery of a high concentration of oxygen (approaching 100 percent), ease of use, and protection from disease transmission. Also, like the resuscitation mask and BVM, the demand valve can deliver oxygen to either breathing or nonbreathing victims.

The disadvantages include higher cost compared with other devices, requirement of a constant source of oxygen, and rapid depletion of a cylinder. In addition, because the oxygen is delivered under higher pressure, complications from overventilation have been reported. This resulted in manufacturers designing demand valves that restricted oxygen flow and installing relief valves to eliminate overinflation when ventilating nonbreathing victims. However, this created another problem. This new, restricted flow demand valve did not always meet the needs of a person in severe respiratory distress. In addition, even with these restrictions, the device should not be used to ventilate nonbreathing children or infants because of the possibility that the device will overinflate the victim.

Some EMS systems have stopped using demand valves. Others use both the newer restricted demand valve for nonbreathing victims and the traditional demand valve for breathing victims. Manufacturers are working to produce one demand valve more appropriate for both breathing and nonbreathing victims.

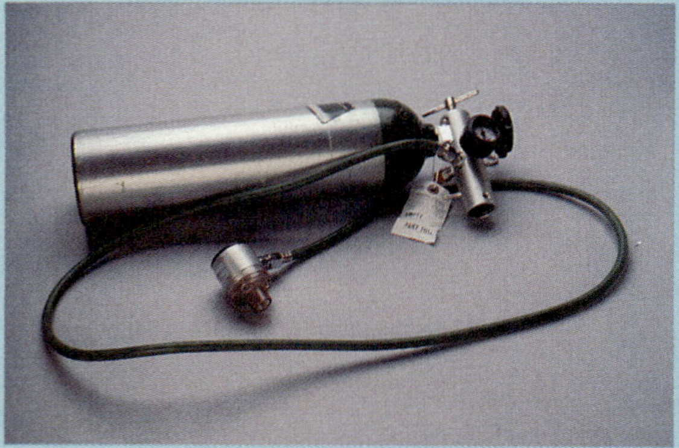

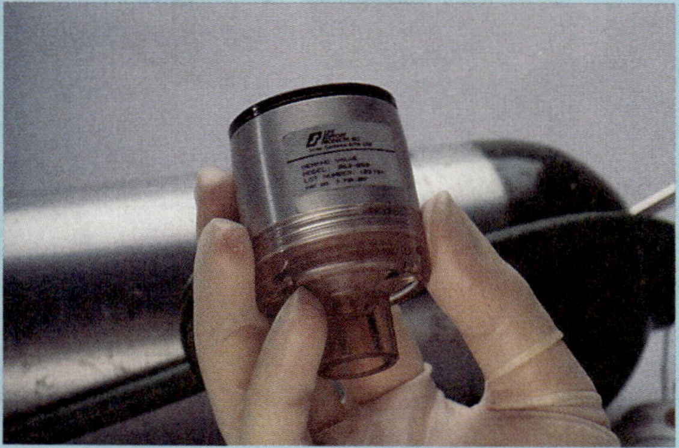

Precautions

When administering oxygen, safety is a primary concern. Remember the following precautions:

- *Do not* operate oxygen equipment around an open flame or sparks. Oxygen causes fire to burn more rapidly.
- *Do not* stand oxygen cylinders upright unless they can be well secured. If the cylinder falls, it could damage the regulator or possibly loosen the cylinder valve.
- *Do not* use grease, oil, or petroleum products to lubricate any pressure regulator parts. Oxygen does not mix with these products, and a severe chemical reaction could cause an explosion.
- Always check to see that oxygen is flowing from the delivery device before placing the device over the person's face.

◆ Clearing the Airway

Sometimes injury or sudden illness results in foreign matter, such as mucus, vomitus, water, or blood, collecting in a victim's airway. The most appropriate initial method of clearing the airway is to roll the person onto his or her side and sweep the obstruction from the mouth. Then reposition the victim and continue providing care.

SUMMARY

Although they are not required, breathing devices can make the emergency care you provide safer, easier, and more effective. The use of supplemental oxygen can relieve pain and breathing discomfort. The resuscitation mask is the most readily available device for the delivery of oxygen, which can significantly increase the oxygen concentration that an ill or injured person needs. Breathing devices can help ventilate a nonbreathing person, and reduce the likelihood of disease transmission.

Breathing devices are appropriate for almost all types of injury or illness in which breathing may be impaired. Knowing how to use these devices will enable you to provide more effective care until more advanced medical personnel arrive.

Use the activities that follow to help you review the material in this booklet.

SELF-ASSESSMENT

Matching

Match each term with its definition. Write its letter on the line in front of the definition.

Terms

- **a** Flowmeter
- **b** Nasal cannula
- **c** Resuscitation mask
- **d** Oxygen cylinder
- **e** Bag-valve-mask (BVM) resuscitator

Definitions

1 ____ A device that regulates oxygen delivery in liters per minute (lpm)

2 ____ An oxygen delivery device best used by two rescuers, because one person may have difficulty keeping the airway open while still maintaining a tight enough seal

3 ____ Used to administer oxygen to a victim who is breathing, but can be ineffective in a victim who has a bad cold

4 ____ A piece of equipment with an internal pressure of approximately 2,000 pounds per square inch

5 ____ A pliable, dome-shaped device that fits over the victim's nose and mouth and is used in giving rescue breathing

True/False

Circle T if the statement is true; circle F if it is false.

1 T F For a proper seal, one rim of the resuscitation mask should be placed between the victim's lower lip and chin.

2 T F One of the advantages of breathing devices is that they allow the rescuer to deliver a higher concentration of oxygen to the victim than simple rescue breathing.

3 T F The oxygen delivery device should be placed over the victim's face before oxygen begins to flow from the device.

4 T F A person who suffers a serious injury can benefit from supplemental oxygen.

5 T F Oxygen should not be administered around open flames or sparks.

Short Answer

Read each statement and write the correct answer or answers in the space provided.

1 The four items of equipment necessary for administration of supplemental oxygen are—

____

____

2 The four safety precautions you should follow when administering oxygen are—

____

____

Multiple Choice

Circle the letter of the best answer.

1 Which is an advantage of using a resuscitation mask to provide artificial ventilation?

- **a** It reduces the volume of air needed to expand the victim's lungs.
- **b** It prevents airway obstruction from occurring as a result of facial injuries.
- **c** It reduces the risk of disease transmission between rescuer and victim.
- **d** All of the above.

2 When using a resuscitation mask, the best way to maintain an open airway is by —

- **a** Tilting the person's head back.
- **b** Lifting the jaw upward.
- **c** Keeping the person's mouth open.
- **d** All of the above.

3 A pressure regulator should not be lubricated with a petroleum product because of the danger of—

- **a** Contamination of the oxygen.
- **b** An explosion.
- **c** Loosening the oxygen cylinder valve.
- **d** Inaccurate readings from the oxygen flowmeter.

4 The O-ring should be placed on the oxygen cylinder—

- **a** After the regulator is in place.
- **b** After you have examined the pressure regulator.
- **c** After you have opened the cylinder for 1 second.
- **d** After you have verified the oxygen flow.

5 Which is a sign of hypoxia?

- **a** Cyanosis
- **b** Unusually slow or fast breathing
- **c** Normal heart rate
- **d** Both a and b

◆ PRACTICE SESSION ◆

Using a Resuscitation Mask for Rescue Breathing

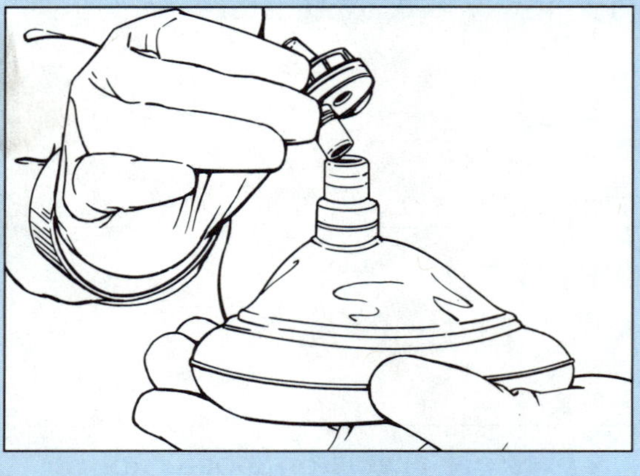

☐ **Assemble the mask**

- ◆ Attach one-way valve to mask.

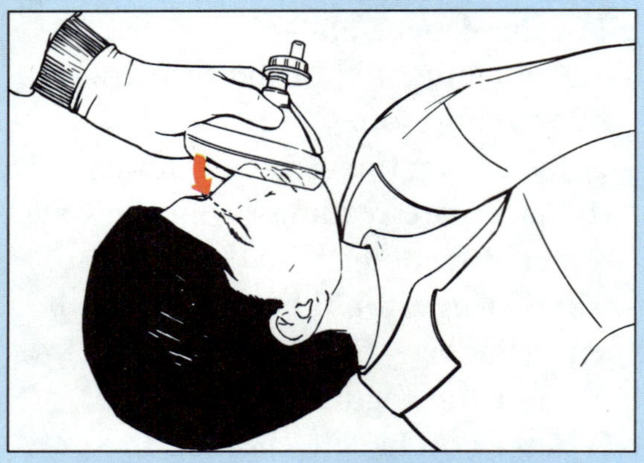

☐ **Position the mask**

- ◆ Kneel behind person's head.
- ◆ Place rim of mask between lower lip and chin.
- ◆ Cover victim's mouth and nose with mask.

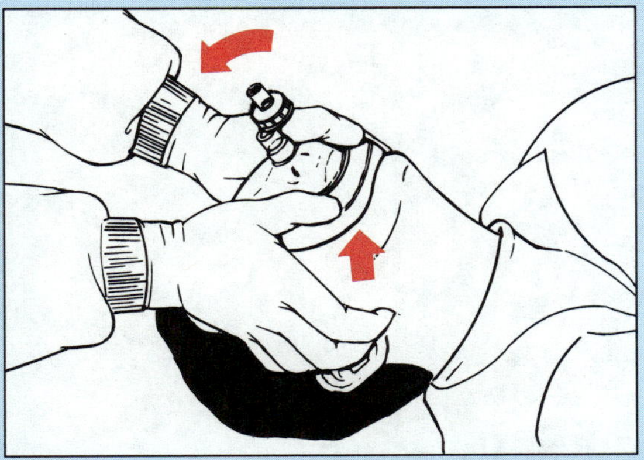

☐ Seal mask and open airway

- Place your thunbs on each side of mask to hold it in place.
- Place fingers of both hands along victim's jawbone.
- Tilt the head back.
- Apply downward pressure with thumbs while lifting the jaw upward with fingers.

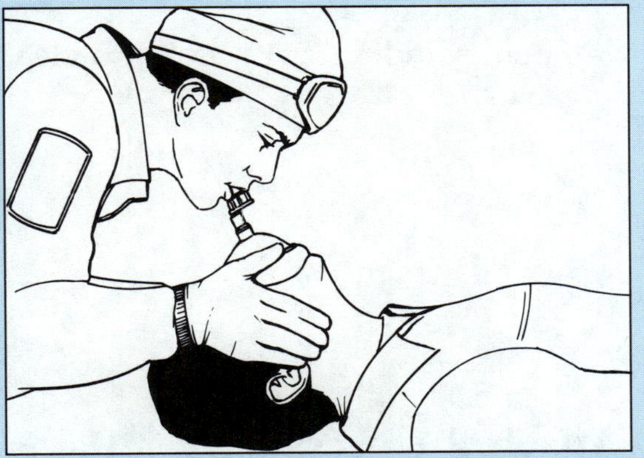

☐ Begin rescue breathing

- Give 1 slow breath about every 5 seconds (once about every 3 seconds for a child or infant).
- Watch chest to see that breaths go in.
- Recheck pulse every minute.

◆ PRACTICE SESSION ◆

Oxygen Delivery

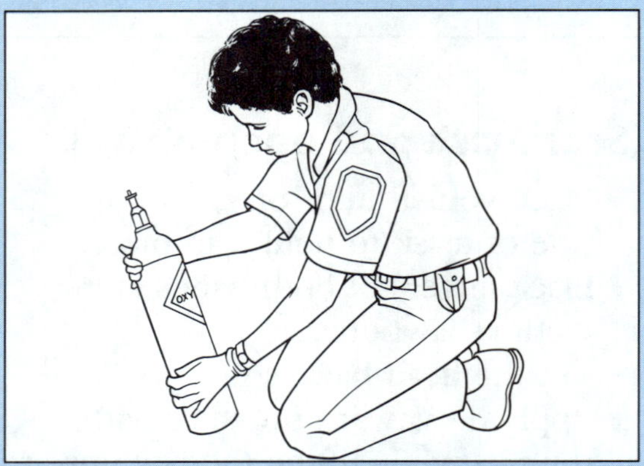

☐ Check the cylinder

- See that label is marked *oxygen.*

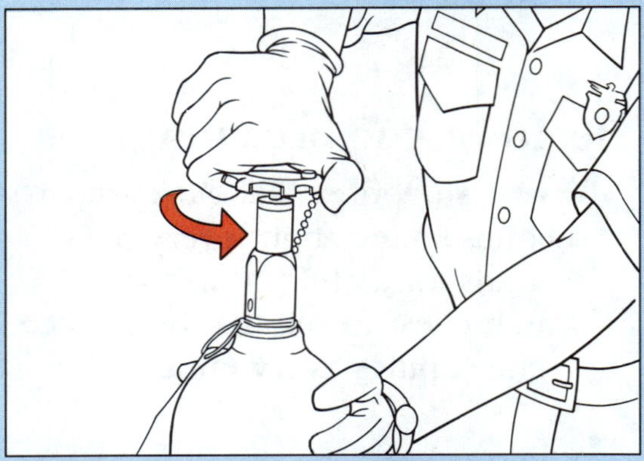

☐ Clear the valve

- Remove protective covering and save plastic gasket.
- Open cylinder for 1 second to clear the valve.

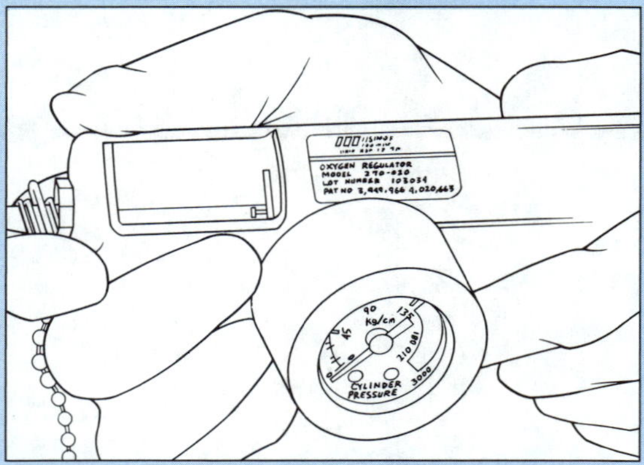

☐ Attach the pressure regulator

- See that it is marked *Oxygen Pressure Regulator.*

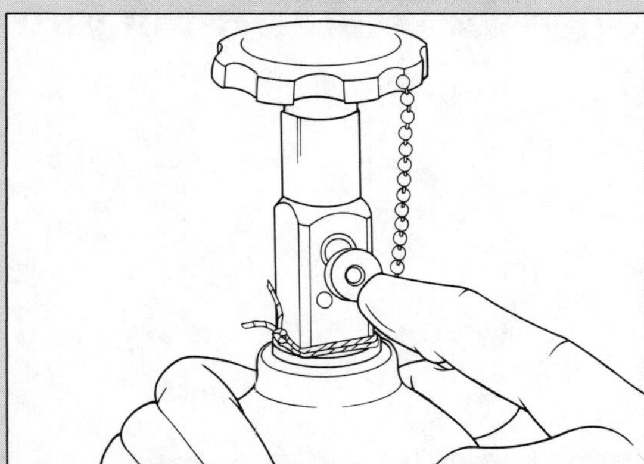

- Put plastic gasket into valve at top of cylinder

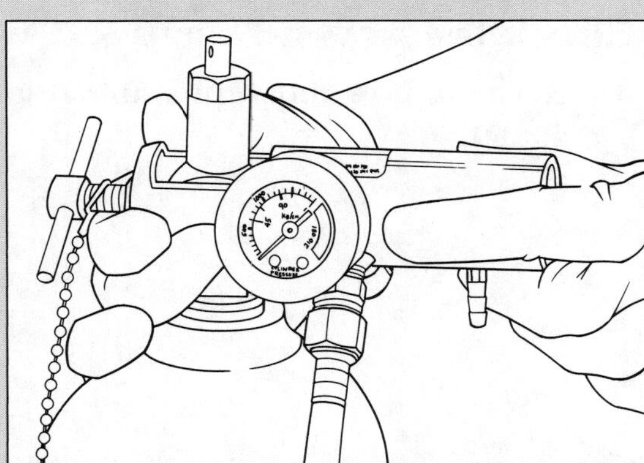

- Place regulator on cylinder.
- Seat the three metal prongs into valve.

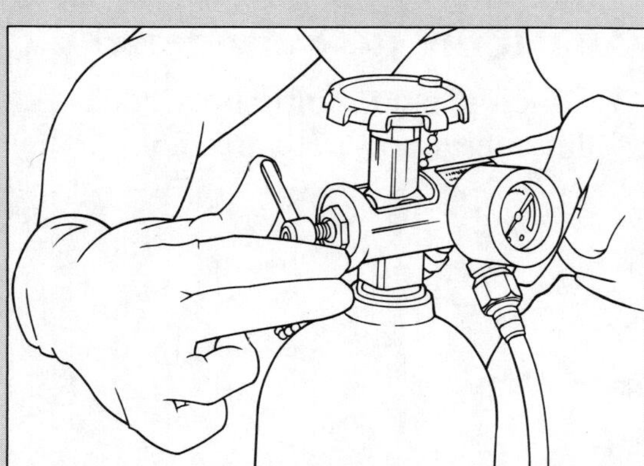

- Hand tighten screw until regulator is snug.

Continued.

◆ PRACTICE SESSION: ◆

Oxygen Delivery—cont'd

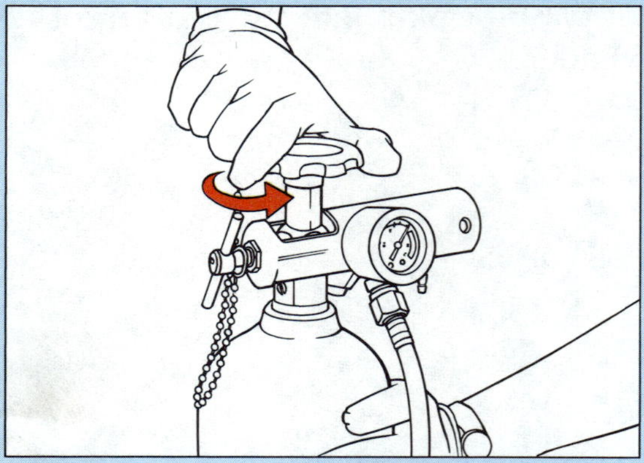

☐ **Open the cylinder 1 full turn**

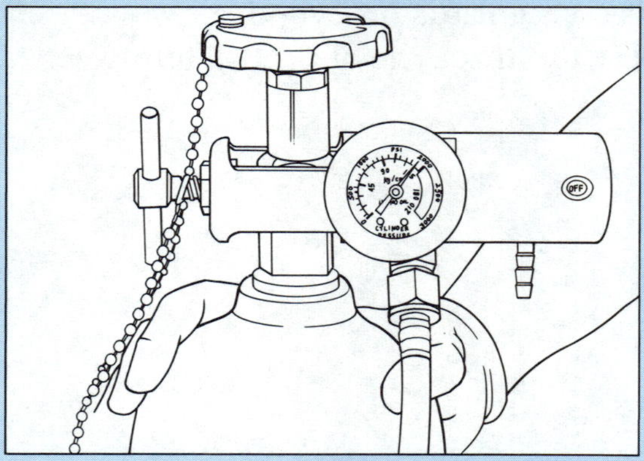

☐ **Check the pressure gauge**

- Determine how much pressure is in cylinder.

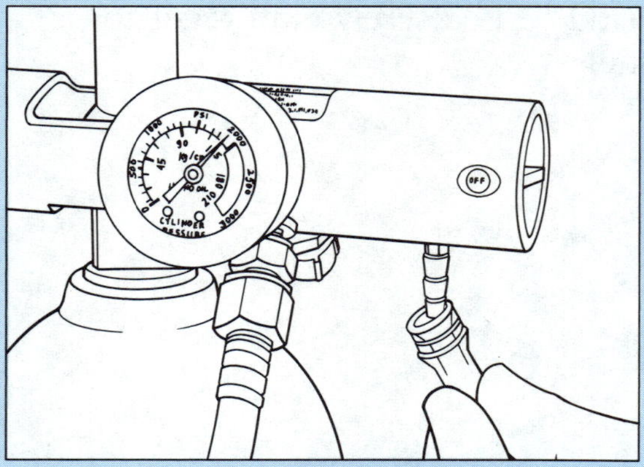

☐ **Attach the delivery device**

- Attach plastic tubing between flowmeter and delivery device.

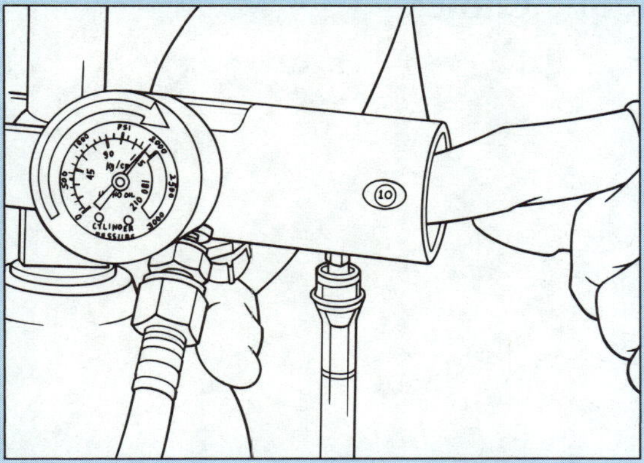

☐ Adjust the flowmeter

- Turn flowmeter to desired flow rate.

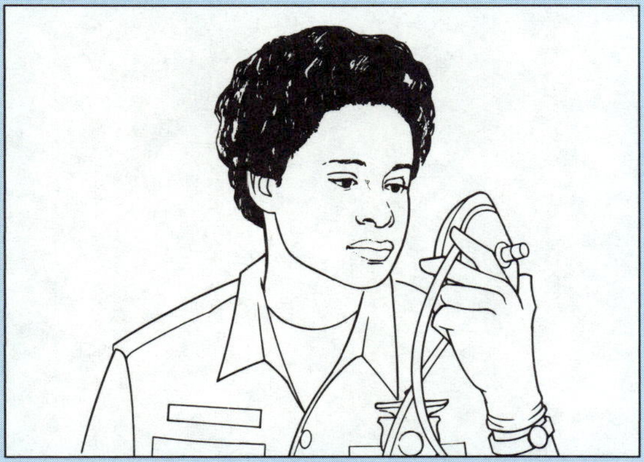

☐ Verify oxygen flow

- Listen and feel for oxygen flow through delivery device.

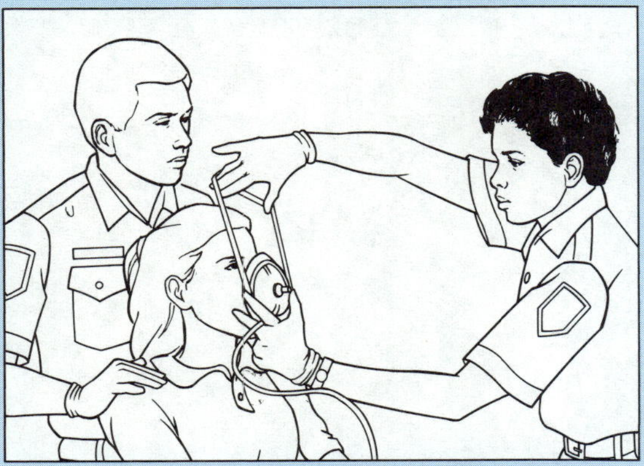

☐ Place the delivery device on victim

Self-Assessment Test Answers

Matching

1. a 2. e 3. b 4. d 5. c

True/False

1. T 2. T 3. F 4. T 5. T

Short Answer

1. Oxygen cylinder; pressure regulator; flowmeter; delivery device
2. Do not operate around open flame or sparks. Do not stand the cylinder upright unless it is secured. Do not use grease, oil, or other petroleum products on the pressure regulator. Always check to see that oxygen is flowing before placing a device on a person's face.

Multiple Choice

1. c 2. d 3. b 4. c 5. a

NOTES

NOTES